The Secrets of Super Strength

T J Oflaherty

DEDICATION

I dedicate this book to my uncle Alfred Howell who started me on my journey into body conditioning and strength training from a very early age and developed my passion for health and fitness.

CONTENTS

Chapter 1

Your motivation and the power of imagination.

1 Why is motivation important in strength training?

Motivation is the number one factor which will keep you on track toward your goals. Nothing more important exists than your motivation. Once you start getting motivated you'll continue moving toward your goal. Motivation is your number one key and driving force in achieving any goal you set. You must really think clearly about what it is you want, why you want it and the price you are prepared to pay to attain it.

You must have your motivation very clearly defined. A focused aim of where you're going and goals which will take you there. Motivation is incredibly powerful, more powerful than any training regime or diet.

Motivation isn't something that pushes you towards your goal. Motivation is something that pulls you toward your goal like iron being pulled towards a magnet. Once your motivation is magnetised you will be immediately pulled towards your goal. You will effortlessly be pulled toward your goal. You will be on course to your destination. Your goal will be an irresistible force. It will be such a strong motivation and so powerful that you will no longer have to force yourself to go to the gym and train.

You must ask yourself what is the reason you want to achieve this goal and then paint a very clear, bright and large picture in your minds eye of exactly what it is you want. The goal must be big and awe inspiring. The bigger the goal, the more powerful the attraction and the more you will be pulled towards it.

The next step is to imagine you have already achieved this goal and you must see yourself in your minds eye succeeding. Once this is done there are very few things on earth that can stop you achieving your goal because YOU are now that irresistible force. Once you believe you are an irresistible force, concepts such as pain, fear and doubt are eliminated from your mind which will allow your mind and body to work in perfect harmony and this is when you will achieve feats of strength beyond your wildest dreams.

The fear of pain or being injured, of failure and doubt are the thoughts and emotions which will curtail any real attempts at even lifting half the weight you can possibly lift. The fear of being judged a failure, the consciousness of people watching you when you lift, the self doubt that you can be strong are the real barriers to becoming super strong. You must convince yourself that you can do it before anyone else can believe it.

The mind has setup many safety systems in the body which over protect the body. A person who potentially is capable of lifting 300 pounds in the bench press but only lift 100 pounds does so because that persons nervous system is telling only 30% of their muscle fibers to lift the weight. *It is only* in times of emergency when the person is under extreme stress that the mind will tell the body to recruit 100% of the muscles to lift the weight.

We have all heard of the mother who has lifted the boot of a car when her child was caught underneath it. Under these circumstances the mind tells the body to send out as much adrenaline and testosterone as the body can handle. This increases blood flow to the muscles, tells the neurons to activate all the muscles and blocks all pain so that the body can be used to its full potential in order to save the child's life. Why can't we perform these feats of amazing strength everyday you may ask. The answer is that the body has many mechanisms to preserve itself and if it used all of theses mechanisms every day the nervous system would burn out.

Strength athletes who do extreme strength lifts cannot continue that level of intensity for more than two weeks. The nervous system cannot handle it. These athletes cycle their training periodically monthly or seasonally and peak between 8 and 12 weeks of pyramid training. There is a fine line between doing just enough to stimulate strength and over doing it which totally shuts down the muscles. Keeping you on the right side of this fine line is what The Secrets of Super Strength is all about.

T J OFlaherty

2 What is the power of imagination?

Imagination is more important than knowledge. **Albert Einstein.**

Knowledge is limited but there is no limit to the power of imagination. Your imagination is directly linked to your subconscious mind and your subconscious drives your most important motivations such as sex, food, warmth and safety. It is the ideas that you plant into your subconscious mind through your imagination that will take your strength to an almost superhuman level.

Lets set the bench mark. Here are the world records of raw powerlifting strength athletes as follows:

Squat: 934 Don Reinhoudt USA 1975 AAU.

Bench Press: 722 Eric Spoto USA 05/19/13

Deadlift: 1015 Benedikt Magnusson ISL 04/02/11.

The lifts stated are about 3 times the amount the average person would normally lift even if they trained on a regular basis but the difference is that these strength athletes know the secrets of super strength.

3 What theories are there in this chapter?

Yoga

Theories in this book are based on sports science and psychology including practices of yoga and martial arts. Why should you rely practices based on yoga and martial arts?

Yoga and martial arts have been developed over thousands of years to around 2800BCE **(p14 Yoga for you - Tara Fraser - Duncan Baird Publishers 2001)**. The benefits are a result of thousands of years of experimentation and observation. Having intense concentration so pure that you are only aware of the object focused on and yourself is one benefit of using the yoga technique called the super conscious state (Samadhi) to give you super strength.

Two other yoga techniques are Asana (posture) which gives you stability and Pranayama (breath control) which strengthens the stability for incredible power transfer through the body. This is similar to the Valsalva Maneuver where the lifter breathes in on the concentric preparation stage of the lift and breathes out on the eccentric execution stage of the lift. This action gives the spine great support.

People who use yoga techniques are able to overcome obstacles such as sickness, lack of mental effort, self doubt, inattention, laziness or fatigue, over indulgence and lack of perseverance. Many yogis are considered contortionists and also perform amazing feats of strength and this is because they practice mental control. This control allows them to endure incredible amounts of pain without feeling or injury. Additional benefits of using yoga techniques are suppleness, stamina, less injuries, posture and detoxing of the body, enhanced digestion and increased awareness.

Super Strength Technique 1

Step1

Before training always sit alone and relax for 5 minutes clearing your mind of all outside thoughts.

Step 2

When your mind is clear breath in slowly through the nose and out of the mouth when doing this imagine you are breathing in energy and you can see this energy entering your body.

Step 3

Imagine this energy is entering different parts of your body starting from your head, then your shoulders and continue this process down your body until you reach your feet. Every breath in and out or (Prana and Apana) is nourishing your body.

Step 4

When you have completed the whole body you will feel your whole body refreshed and bursting with latent energy. At this point you will feel an irresistible urge to train and unleash that energy. This is the first secret to super strength.

Yoga poses:

Basic yoga poses should be used as a light stretch and warm up before touching any weights. Example poses include Sun salutation and for warm downs you can do half sun salutations.

Martial arts

"The term tai chi refers to the yin-yang symbol prevalent in Chinese culture, more commonly known as the "hard" and "soft" sign- the opposites coming together".**(p195 The Ultimate Book of Martial Arts Fay Goodman, Hermes House 2003).**

The benefits of a martial art such as Fa jing which is from Tai Chi Chuan is to issue power from close range incorporating the whole body into one unit. To develop super strength you must have a body that can focus all of its power into one movement and Tai Chi Chuan is an art form which will help you to develop that ability. It is your sensitivity rather than your brute force that will allow you to develop super strength because the more you can feel a weight or resistance, the more you can recruit muscle fibers to contract. Likewise the less sensitive you are to resistance, the less muscle you can recruit to contract against that resistance. Tai Chi Chuan aims to allow the practitioner to relax in order for the body to become more efficient. When the body is efficient it can then apply maximum force. For every action there is an equal and opposite reaction. For the body to be able to control this reaction to force it must be relaxed in the appropriate places. One of the greatest exponents of martial arts was Bruce Lee. He was famous for, amongst other things, the one inch punch with which he devastated his opponents. By moving a mere inch but using his body weight he produced massive amounts of power. He did this by focusing his mind to punch beyond the target and by combining breathing, balance, speed and perfect technique.

Bruce Lee was an advocate of a form of weight training called isometrics. When most martial artists believed weight training would make you slow Bruce Lee was pumping iron and developing super strength.

Super Strength Technique 2

Step 1

Before lifting a heavy weight you should gently stretch the muscle you are about to train. This action will create an elastic effect in the golgi tendon and the muscles and the muscles will involuntarily contract. This contraction will give your strength a boost of invisible power enervated naturally from the body's own elasticity. This is called Stretch Reflex. When you do one thing to the body the body attempts to keep its yin - yang balance and it reacts in the opposite way.

Step 2

You must imagine yourself lifting the weight before you lift it. This action subconsciously makes the mind think it has already lifted the weight, the action also fires motor neurons even though no weight had been lifted. The mental technique prepares you neurologically and mentally for the task ahead.

Step 3

This is the most difficult part and the reason why you must really work hard on training the mind to focus. What you must do before lifting the weight is to tense the whole body very quickly this will have the effect of relaxing the body immediately afterwards. The result is that body will be relaxed enough to control the descent of the weight during the stretch phase of the movement and the body will be toned enough to react to the stress of the weight for the ascent of the lift.

Developing the above techniques based on Yoga and Martial arts will give you the mental focus techniques for power which were developed and refined over thousands of years. What you are doing is subconsciously reconfiguring your threshold for pain, releasing testosterone and adrenaline and creating self fulfilling prophesies by destroying fears and doubts. How many people do you know meditate, use visualisation techniques and use martial arts philosophies before they lift a weight? Probably none, simply because they are not motivated enough to achieve the goal of becoming super strong. The price tag is not taking drugs, nor drinking every supplement or miracle herb on the market, the price tag is being dedicated enough to making your mind super strong. Once you have a strong mind, the body follows suite.

Self Hypnosis

Hypnosis is direct control or suggestion of the subconscious mind and this according to Paul Mckenna "contains all your wisdom, memories and intelligence; it is your source of creativity. It regulates body maintenance and automatic processes like breathing, blood circulation and tissue regeneration." **The Hypnotic World of Paul Mc Kenna, Boston 1993**. Psychology affects your mental attitude and mental attitude has an incredible affect on your strength. **J A Hadfield in the Psychology of power** discovered when testing 3 men that the subjects grip strength was almost 50% stronger when they were given positive thoughts about their strength level. The conclusion of the point is that if you believe it, you can achieve it. Or rather if you believe it enough then you can achieve it.

Super Strength Technique 3

This is the most unusual and most embarrassing technique of the three

Super Strength Techniques however it is this technique which will give you the best results. To be extraordinary you must be prepared to do things that are out of the ordinary.

Step 1

Watch a strength athlete you that admire and want to emulate.

Step 2

Relax into a trance like state for which you need refer to the Yoga technique of relaxation but instead of breathing normally you hold your breath for 2 seconds before moving onto a different body part. When you finally reach the feet you should be completely relaxed.

Step 3

Imagine the person in from of you and build the picture of them as clearly and big as possible. Add sounds and colours and feelings to the picture.

Step 4

Ask this person to help you and imagine them obliging and offering to help you.

Step 5

Now walk behind the person and walk into their body and imagine you see through their eyes and hear through their ears, attempt to walk around in their body in your imagination.

Step 6

Find out what its like to be in the role models body and try doing something that you want to do while in their body such as imagining lifting a certain amount of weight. Then remember how it feels when you lifted that weight.

Step 7

Step out of your role models body and thank him or her for their help and remember what you experienced.

Step 8

Return to normal waking consciousness and just wait to see the results of this one!

4 How do you motivate yourself?

When you have established a powerful aim, the next step is to create short easily attainable goals which take you towards your aim. These goals should in themselves offer you rewards so that your motivation is spiked every time you reach a goal. You should celebrate every time you reach a goal and that is how you motivate yourself and stay motivated.

Your aim and goals must be SMART (specific, measurable, achievable, results orientated and target driven). If your goal is to bench press 50 kilo grams more in the bench press in 1 month. The goal would be specific but not achievable based on normal experience although that is not to say it is impossible.

A SMART way to achieve the aim of bench pressing 50 kilos would be to measure how much the average person would normally improve each week. It is possible to improve 1 kilogram gradually on a weekly basis. This allows you to measure 50 weeks and allows you to see that it is a reasonable aim and goal. It is reasonable for most beginners to increase their bench press weight within a year by 50 kilos or more. It is even possible for Intermediate strength trainers who have conditioned bodies to improve by 50 kilograms but it is unusual for advanced trainers to do this within a year because at an advanced level it is likely you have already tried most of the training techniques, had many injuries and are not still as motivated as the beginner or intermediate. That said there are power lifters who have improved their bench press by 50 kilos in one year by changing; their grip on the bar, their diet, their rest periods, their training partners, their gym and most important of all, changing their mental attitude.

5 Which visualisation techniques do you use?

The visualisation technique number 3 really works for the author and many high level athletes and can fire your imagination. It may sometimes takes a few days or even up to a month to find your ideal role model but when you do find that mental image then it will take your strength to the next level.

6 What is my strength potential?

The human potential is unlimited. In the 1950s scientist believed that if man ran faster than 10 seconds in the hundred meter sprint that it would create so much pressure that the athletes head would explode. Scientists also believed that no man could run the mile faster than 4 minutes. Time and time again science attempts to limit human potential with barriers and athletes continually break these barriers.

Human beings are not static entities they are actually adaptive beings which respond to stress and become stronger and faster. Humans have gone beyond natural selection and are now engineering their own bodies and minds through progressive training systems. There is no limitation to your potential apart from the one in your mind. Everyone believed going under the 4 minute mile was impossible, apart from Roger Bannister. Belief is everything.

7 How do you stick to goals?

It is not enough to just set goals and visualise, you must also be held accountable for your goals. Tell people that you are aiming for a certain goal and update them on a regular basis about it. This action creates a partnership of accountability and reassures you that your goals are important not only to you but others who want to see you succeed.

8 Why is self esteem important?

The author started training because he was very skinny as a result of being under nourished as a child He wanted to improve his self esteem and obtain some respect amongst his peer group. He also was motivated by the Charles Atlas advertisements in comic books. Many people start training with weights not only to build bulk and become big and strong but also as a response to being bullied, negative body image, a need for acceptance from their peer group, and to imitate their role models.

9 Why is a support structure important?

A support structure is like a fan or cheer leading team who push you when you going through the weak times and when you are losing motivation.

The support structure could be a family member, a friend or a training partner or trainer. If you have no one you know to support you then you could take the daring step of uploading your video progress on social media and let the public push and motivate you to being accountable to your goals and aims.

10 Why are mantras and quotes important for motivation?

Never underestimate the power of words and the effect they have on your mental and physical health. Telling yourself everyday that you will achieve your goals and believing what you say to yourself is essential. Mantras are incredibly powerful tools for creating self fulfilling prostheses.

These positive words release the power of the endocrine system which releases hormones that boosts your bodies' capacity for amazing strength.

Here are some quotes from the worlds most famous body builder who incidentally started out as a power lifter.

Arnold Schwarzenegger.

"Dig deep down and ask yourself, who do you want to be. Not what but who you want to be. Figure out for yourself what makes you happy."

"Trust yourself, no matter what or how anyone else thinks."

"Don't be afraid to fail. Don't be afraid to make decisions."

"You never want to fail because you didn't work hard enough."

The Secrets of Super Strength

Chapter 2

The Science of Strength Training

1 How strong is the human body?

With around 208 bones in the human body and these bones being able to take a pressure of about 450 kilograms **(The human body- a family reference book- Cotton and Adam - Paragon Publishing 2012)** this means that with the extra shock absorbing qualities tendons, ligaments, muscle, fat and water, the body can support the pressure a several tons. Bone tissue consists mainly of calcium and proteins such as collagen and elastin giving them flexibility and elasticity.

GUINNESS BOOK OF RECORDS

At the time of writing this book the world deadlift record was 1015 lbs. held by BENEDIKT MAGNUSSON. This gives you an idea of the enormous strength potential people have.

2 How many muscles and cells are there in the body?

There are 650 skeletal muscles also known as voluntary muscles. There are a billion cells in the human body and one cell alone can divide up to 50 times before dying. There are 9 systems in the body, these consist of; circulatory, skeletal, nervous, lymphatic, muscular, digestive, urinary, respiratory and endocrine. More important than the muscular system is the circulatory system because this is driven by the heart which via the blood fluid provides nutrients for the whole body. All these systems must work in harmony. Over developing one system without considering the balance of the others will in the long term will hold back your attainment of super strength. A very important system is the endocrine system because this is formed by the glands in the body. They send out the hormones which control growth and metabolism and this system is heavily influenced by emotions. Emotions are influenced by your belief systems and your diet which is an area we will cover in later chapters.

The muscles are attached to tendons and tendons are attached to ligaments which connect to bone. Sometimes ligaments directly connect bone to bone. Most joints are synovial joints which mean they are versatile and lubricate. This lubrication is called synovial fluid. Synovial fluid acts a shock absorber and stops the bones rubbing against each other which can cause degenerative diseases such as tendonitis and arthritis. This is why it is incredibly important to warm up before any exercise even if the exercise is with light weights.

3 What determines strength?

Muscle fiber is made up of 5 main areas (myofibril, sarcomere, actin myosin filaments and titin)and it is important to remember these as it will give you a focus of the effect training and diet will have on these areas.

The nervous system tells the muscles to contract and calcium is released into the muscle cell which allows actin and myosin to rub against each other. This shortens the muscle and thus pulls the body to create movement. What is fascinating is that actin and myosin is required for the release of calcium to work. Bones are heavily composed of calcium and this should indicate that calcium should be a major factor in your diet considering its influence on your bone and muscle strength.

Determiners of strength vary widely. Here are 6 factors that determine strength:

1 Bone length,

2 muscle length, height (ectomorph, endomorph or mesomorph)

3 muscle type, (fast twitch and slow twitch)

4 natural muscle, tendon and ligament strength

5 mental attitude

6 diet.

Of the 6 factors that influence strength only mental attitude and diet are under your full control. Children who do a lot of exercise can influence their bone and muscle length and even muscle type but once they have reached maturity and their bones have fossilised there is little you can do to increase these factors. Therefore your mental attitude and your diet are two things to which you must give 100% of your energy.

Your diet will determine the natural strength of your ligaments and tendons. This will in turn determine the strength of your muscle contraction. Even someone who has strong muscles will soon become injured if they don't have strong enough tendons and ligaments to support the stress and pressure they incur from lifting very heavy weights.

Bone length will influence how much weight you can lift because the law of physics determines that to move the same weight for a longer distance requires more force. But there is an advantage to having long levers in that the power generated by the longer lever will be explosive and release more power. This is why tall high jumpers, long jumpers and sprinters can propel themselves great distances in a shorter timer (= Power) when strength training is added to their training program.

T J OFlaherty

Chapter 3

Your Body Type

Most people are divided into 3 body types:

A ectomorph

Slim build with long limbs, wide shoulders and have short torsos.

B endomorph

The opposite of the ectomorph in that they have wide hips, a higher percentage of body fat, longer torso but short limbs.

C mesomorph

Thick build with short arms and legs like the endomorph but a lower body fat percentage and quite muscular.

Naturally the mesomorph with the muscular build has the most strength because of leverage and muscle advantage however something interesting happens after intense training. The endomorph catches with the mesomorph because of their ability to absorb nutrients and convert them into good fat (poly unsaturated) which help release growth hormone! Even more surprising is the effect of training on the ectomorph. The ectomorphs' ability to develop strength is incredible. This person can develop amazing strength due to 2 factors: 1 they have long levers which indicate long muscle length and 2 they have a fast metabolism which means that they can consume large amounts protein, carbohydrate and fat which can develop very strong muscles, tendons and ligaments.

4 What are fast and slow twitch muscles?

Fast and Slow twitch muscle. This is where most research has been done and answers the question as to whether athletes are born or made.

In the book **Powerlifting** by Austin and Mann, muscle fiber types decides whether a person of 82 kilograms can lift 700 pounds in the bench press or can squat 800 pounds. The number of fast twitch fibers dictates to a large extent your level of a strength and speed.

In **Serious Strength Training** by Bompa and Di Pasquale the muscles are divided and three types and 2 general types of muscle fiber. There are fast and slow twitch described as type IIA and IIX(some journals describe Iix as type IIB).

Slow twitch: type 1

The slow twitch muscles are known as type 1A. Slow twitch fibers are the fibers which provide you with long term energy for activities that are repetitive or constant.

Energy that carries on for periods longer than 40 seconds continuously can be considered slow twitch. There are different accounts of how long certain types of fibers can perform for. Activities that last for hours can be considered type I fibers which are small, slow, red in colour and have a high resistance to fatigue, a high michondrial and capillary density. Their energy source is triglycerides which mean it is made from a glycerol and three fatty acids. This is important to know this when training because the energy sources decides how effective your training will be. The triglycerides enable the movement of fat and blood glucose from the liver for energy.

A great advantage for people who predominantly have type 1 slow twitch fiber is that they can use lactic acid as an energy source. Lactic acid is a by product of exercise and so the energy has a continuous cycle.

Fast Twitch: type 2

These are the most diverse muscle fibers in that they have a hybrid of performance properties.

type 2A

These are red in colour contract moderately fast, medium in size and good for long term anaerobic power. The duration of the performance is normally less than 30 minutes. Its energy source is creatine phosphate glycogen. Creatine is product of energy found mainly in red meat, but also in eggs and fish.

type 2X

These are fast, large and have intermediate levels of resistance to fatigue. The muscle is best used for short term anaerobic work for less than 5 minutes. The power produced is high and the michondrial density is medium although the capillary density is low. Hence the development for increasing endurance is limited. These muscles use ATP, Creatine phosphate and a small amount of glycogen.

type 2B

The final type of muscle fiber is what creates elite strength and power athletes. This fiber contracts very fast is very larger but has a low resistance to fatigue and is best used for short term energy, less than 1 minute in length. Its power output is very high but its michondrial and capillary density is low so there is very little development possibilities for endurance because it has low glycolic capacity. The advantages however are that it feeds on ATP and creatine phosphate.

Chapter 4

Foods that are high in protein, carbohydrates and vitamins and minerals. Specifically foods that contain vitamin D, calcium and zinc combined with iodine will help promote growth in people who have not yet reached puberty and in their early twenties. For mature adults most diary products especially eggs and milk will promote growth. Vegetables from tropical climates like yams and green bananas will stimulate growth hormones in the body.

Your Diet

Of the six things that contribute to strength the most important is your diet.

The adage that you are what you eat is only true up to a point. Yes, If you eat lots of fat and don't exercise, you become fat, but if you eat lots of protein and carbohydrates and don't exercise you also become fat. It is possible to have a high fat low protein low carbohydrate diet and still become strong and toned. The question is what type of fats are you eating, when are you eating them and what type of training are you doing. You cannot absorb large amounts of protein, fats and carbohydrates without the necessary vitamins and minerals which help to digest this food. If you do then you may end up with a bloated stomach because you are unable to breakdown the large amounts of food. Strength training will help build muscle and shape but it will also produce a large bloated stomach if the right nutrients are not digested with the foods.

Water

Most weight trainers would probably say the number one most important nutrient to increase in your diet for strength is protein. Wrong! the most important nutrient is water.

Protein only makes up 30 % of the body where as water makes up almost 70%. And most of muscle content is actually water and not muscle. A 2% level of dehydration can lead to a 5% dip in performance. That 5% dip in performance may be the reason why you haven't improved in your training. It may be the reason why you are not reaching your goals.

Water is the most important nutrient, because without this, nothing else can function. You also need to drink enough water because if you don't the body digests food slower.

The body requires water for nearly all of its chemical reactions and if there is not enough water then it slows down and one effect is bloating of the stomach, puffiness around the eyes and a dry mouth.

Protein

There is much debate about how many grams of protein you should take. One thing is for certain, if you don't consume enough protein, your attempts at becoming super strong will come to nothing and all of your efforts in the gym will be wasted.

How much protein should you consume per day? Many articles suggest you consume 2 grams of protein per kilo of your body weight. If that is the case and you weight 100kg, you would have to consume 200g of protein which is equal to approximately 6 tins of tuna steak per day. For a super strength athlete this amount of protein is not unusual. Although how much of that protein can you absorb? is a much more important question. The following explanations will give you a background what your protein is and what it does for you.

Protein is the building block of all muscle, tendon and ligaments in the body. It is made up of strands of amino acids and performs a variety of tasks such as replicating DNA, transporting molecules around the body and is essential in every process within the cells. When protein is digested it is broken down into amino acids. Protein also allows for a positive nitrogen balance which is assists growth because it puts you into an anabolic state. The amino acids build the myosin and actin which are responsible for moving the body by sliding against each other which is the muscle contraction.

After vigorous anaerobic training has taken place the body can absorb much higher levels of protein in order to over compensate for the damage done to the muscles during training and build stronger and bigger muscles.

Protein high foods

From the highest % out of 100g to the lowest these include whey protein isolate with a protein content of 90g, whey protein concentrate which is harder to digest at 89g, soy protein at 80g, and then the solid food of beef steak at 34g, chicken great at 31g, salmon at 25g and canned tuna at 19g. Of the vegetables soy bean is very high at 12g per 100g.

Fats

These are classified as saturated or unsaturated and can be further sub classified as mono saturates and poly unsaturated. the saturated fat generally is solid at room temperature and the unsaturated fats are liquid at room temperature such as olive oil.

The benefits of unsaturated fats are many. These include balanced hormone levels, immune protection, normal growth and healthy functioning of the endocrine system (the glands of the body).

Omega 3 and omega 6 are very good examples of nutrients you can get out of unsaturated fats that can help lower cholesterol. Whereas saturated fats also called trans-fats will do the opposite and raise cholesterol.

Carbohydrates

Carbohydrates are a form of sugar and classified as mono saccharides, disaccharides, or polysaccharides depending on the number of sugar chains they contain. Food such as rice, pasta, bread and grain contain large amounts of carbohydrate. Poly saccharides are considered complex carbohydrates because of the number of sugar chains in them.

For many years it was thought that simple carbohydrates were absorbed quickly and complex carbohydrates were slowly absorbed. It is now found that some complex carbohydrates can be absorbed just as quickly as simple ones. The carbohydrate is partially converted into glucose and this stimulates the production of insulin.

Fiber

Fiber is a carbohydrate (or polysaccharide) that humans find difficult to absorb because they lack a certain enzyme to absorb the cellulose within the fiber.

There are two types of finer, soluble and insoluble. Whole grains, fruit and vegetables are good sources of fiber and offer many health benefits such as reducing gastrointestinal problems. Certain fibers can reduce the insulin spikes and reduce type 2 diabetes.

Minerals

Minerals are the chemical elements required by all living beings. These can be subdivided into macro minerals and trace minerals.

Macro minerals

These are essential and often play a role as electrolytes.

The main minerals include: calcium, chloride ions, magnesium (which builds bone and increases alkalinity), phosphorus, (needed for energy production), potassium for heart and nerve health, sodium which is a very common electrolyte (note excessive sodium reduces your calcium and magnesium which can lead to osteoporosis.

Sulphur which is needed to absorb three essential amino acids which help growth and repair of hair, skin, nails, liver and pancreas.

Trace minerals

These are required in trace amounts to help enzymes function. They include, cobalt for absorbing vitaminB12, copper, chromium for sugar metabolism, Iodine for the thyroid, iron for hemoglobin and other proteins, Manganese for oxygen, Molybdenum, Nickel, Selenium an antioxidant, Vanadium and Zinc which is needed by several enzymes and is extremely important for raising testosterone levels.

Vitamins

Vitamins are considered essentials for good health and not having a diet with enough vitamin, A,D and C can lead to scurvy, osteoporosis and impaired immune system disorders such as premature ageing, cancer and poor psychological health.

Phytochemicals

These are trace chemicals found in colourful fruits and vegetable such as black berries. They are known to have polyphenol antioxidants. These include; Zeaxanthin , beta- cryptoxanthin helps against arthritis, lycopene for cancer treatment and Lutein for protection of the eyes from cataracts.

In the following chapters you will read about super intensive training regimes which will test your determination and tolerance to pain but if you ensure that you are taking high protein, the necessary amount of carbohydrates and all the essential vitamins and minerals with every meal then you ability to achieve super levels of strength will be greatly increased.

The quick fix for many strength athletes is to take prohibited/illegal drugs such as steroids or growth hormones. What these athletes have chosen to do is ignore the fact that most vitamins are steroids and that if they combined them in the right quantities over the long term they would become super strong without the side effects of the illegal or prohibited drugs. The reader should bare in mind that building strength is part and parcel of building a strong healthy body. Taking drugs will give you a strong body but it won't be a healthy body, especially in the long term.

Everybody has different nutritional needs and it would be inappropriate to guide everyone to take the same nutrients. What is more important is that everyone has a balanced diet of fats, proteins, carbohydrates, vitamins, minerals and phytochemicals (colourful fruits and vegetables). How much of each food type you should eat depends on the lifestyle you lead. A marathon runner would have a different diet to a sprinter, a powerlifter different to an olympic weightlifter, a body builder different to an all-round fitness athlete.

What foods and nutrients should you take to get strong?

There are many ways to answer this question. First, which foods have you eaten in the past and the following day you felt really strong and energetic. If you can answer this question, you already know which foods work for developing your strength.

The best way of finding out how much food and which type of foods help you get strong is by testing different amounts of protein on a daily basis. Try eating a balanced diet and note how much protein you eat. Then make an extra note of how you feel a few hours after the meal. Do you feel full and satisfied or do you feel that even though your stomach is full you feel there is something missing and not quite right in your body. It this is the case maybe your diet is deficient in protein, carbohydrate, or fruit and vegetables (vitamins and minerals). The next day eat the same meal but more protein and see how you feel, the following day more carbohydrate and the next more vegetables.

By this process of adding and experimenting, you will find the missing link in your diet and be more confident of getting amazing strength gains from your training.

The following chapters will cover training programs for different types and levels of strength trainers it will also cover the diet you need to take to help you achieve your goals.

The Secrets of Super Strength

5 Strength training for a beginner

It should be made clear from the outset of the training programs in this book are not body building programs, nor a crossfit,. This book is for people who seriously want to improve their level of strength. You will not find 100s of exercises for building mass nor ultra high rep training regimes. You will not see lots of exercises. There are a maximum of 4 compound or main exercises that are supplemented by 6-7 core stability exercises. They will not build great size but they will build incredible all-round strength if you stick to the program and take in the right nutrients.

I'm a beginner, how do I get strong quickly?

A beginner in the world of strength training must start with a strong motivation to begin and continue training because most people who start a new activity quit after a few weeks or months after initiation.

Whatever your motivation, it is essential for the beginner to have some guidance from a person who is a qualified and/or experienced strength trainer. Beginners are very often prone to wanting to build muscles fast and want to get strong quickly. They often want to compete with other trainers in the gym in how strong they are in particular on the bench press and arm exercises. This is to be avoided because competition without knowledge of safe lifting technique and knowledge of how often and how hard to train will quickly lead to frustration and even injury.

The first step to becoming strong.

It must be pointed out that the purpose of the beginner routine is to create a foundation for building super strength. You will not become super strong in 9 weeks although you will definitely become much stronger. It is very important that you start by using the **Super Strength Techniques** that are at the beginning of this book before starting any of the training sessions.

This program will develop core stability, strengthen your bones, tendons, ligaments, immune system and raise your hormone levels. Doing body weight exercises. This will give you a good measure of how strong you are pound for pound. It will also give you good coordination and balance for lifting free weights.

The following program should be done every other day, three times a week e.g. Monday, Wednesday and Friday with the weekend off for rest. It should be done for three weeks.

This three week preparation is to ready the body for the stresses and strains of heavier training, lactic acid recovery and to raise the testosterone and adrenalin levels to boost strength.

The short rest periods and force impact star jumps and burpees will activate the fast twitch muscles for the power and explosive strength needed in the later stages of training.

The deep breathing allows for full use of the controlling air in the lungs to create stability when lifting weights. The stretching helps in two ways. Firstly, it reduces lactic acid in the muscles and secondly it lengthens the muscle which increases the muscles potential to produce power.

The intensity of the exercise should be moderate but you should not be straining to do any of the exercises. You just need to feel the movements and workup a slight sweat.

If you can't complete a full press up or pull up, don't beat your self up over it just do half reps until you feel slight discomfort. Please note, you must not strain during the exercise. What you need to do is just feel the movement and build up a sweat.

The diet in this section should be mainly fruits and vegetables with not more than your normal amount of protein e.g. protein with eat meal. If you train and after your meal feel unsatisfied, then maybe add a bit more protein such as half a tin of tuna and extra egg or milk and cheese.

Your best friend the Squat Rack and Power Rack

Your best friend for strength training are the squat rack and power rack because are not only used for the squat but also can be used for the bench press and deadlift. Which saves you from potential serious injury and gives you the confidence to go full out on a set because of the safety measures on these racks.

Spotters

Spotter are normally people who you may or may not know who you ask to pass the weight to you and who is supposed to ensure that if you are attempting to do an extra repetition they will offer a little assistance and also protect you if you are in danger of injuring yourself.

From the authors 30 years experience of training, most injuries are caused by spotters who have done one of the following things:

xliv

A: literally thrown or dropped the weight onto the trainer,

B: walked away immediately after giving the weight to the trainer.

C: not followed the instructions of the trainer.

D: mistimed the passing over of the weight to the trainer.

E: volunteered to spot when they didn't know what the trainer had asked them to do. Here is a scenario:

Trainer: Can you pass me the weight for 2 negative reps and lift the weight up when it touches my chest?

Spotter: Yes I can do that no problem.

The spotter proceeds to pass a weight to the trainer in the bench press of 120% of the trainers' maximum bench press because the trainer is working on negative (eccentric) strength. However when the weight touches the trainer's chest, the spotter goes into auto pilot and tries to get the trainer to do a forced rep. A forced rep with a weight that is 120% of the trainers maximum weight. The trainer is saying lift the weight, take it. The spotter is saying come on one more rep you can do it!

Conclusion: The trainer ends up tearing a pectoral muscle and dislocates his shoulder.

Clearly the spotter didn't know what they were doing but the fault is also the trainers because when you put your safety in someone else's hands you should know that they are experienced in what you are asking them to do and confident that they understand the instructions.

When it comes to strength training, you need very experienced trainers to spot you if you are using advanced training techniques such as negatives, speed training, polymetrics and maximum high sets volume training

WEEK 1 - 3

Body weight exercises	Repetitions and sets	Rest
Sit ups	10 x 2	30 seconds
Press ups (on knees then full)	10 x 2	10 seconds
Squats (half then full)	20 x 2	30 seconds
Star jumps and burpees	25 x 2	1 minute
close grip pull ups (half then full)	5 x 2	1 minute
Skipping	Varied x1	5 minutes
Stationary Bike ride	10 minutes x1	1 minute
Deep breathing slowly (through the nose and out the mouth)	10 x 2	Varied
Stretching back, legs, chest and stomach	5	N/A

WEEK 4 - 6

In week 4 you are now ready for a weight training session with machines and free weights. You have adjusted to using your muscles and coordinating them in power movements and built up a slight tolerance to the lactic acid that you get when exercising anaerobically. Now you have to adjust to using free weights and machine weights for building a foundation for super strength.

The following program is to be followed twice a week e.g. Monday and Thursday with Friday and the weekend to rest. It focuses more on the technique and stability of the strength and power movements.

In order to create this strength stability you must start to consume more protein than normal. 1 gram of protein to 1 kilogram of body weight. This amount is less than most body building and weight lifting journals suggest but will be dramatically much more than the average person who is not used to weight training. At this level exercises should not be a strain. You need to just focus on correct slow movement of the bar and breathing with the movement.

Each exercise should start with an empty bar and 10 kilograms should be added to the bar until the bar feels slightly heavy but you are able to do 10 repetitions. Then for the following sets keep adding 10 kilograms. When you know what your strength level is then you apply that starting weight to week 7.

STRENGTH TRAINING PROGRAM WEEK 4- 6

Weight exercises	Repetitions and sets	Rest
Squats (high bar squats)	10 x 1, 8 x 1, 5 x 3 sets	1 minutes
Power cleans	10 x 1, 7 x 1, 5 x 3 sets	2 minutes
Overhead presses	10 x1, (7 x 3 sets)	2 minutes
Pull downs	10 x 1, 8 x 3 sets	1 minute
Sit ups	10 x 3 sets	1 minute
Leg raises	10 x 3 sets	1 minute
Stationary Bike ride	15 minutes x1	1 minute
Deep breathing	10 x 2 sets	varied
Stretching back, legs, chest and stomach	5	N/A

WEEK 7 - 9

This is where as a beginner you will really experience your first taste from the intense pain of weight training.

There was a six week introduction which eased you into developing stability and fitness for strength, now comes the first real strength workout which should leave you with some heavy lactic acid build up and muscle soreness for a couple of days after training. Because of the increased intensity this program should be done every 4 days e.g. Monday and Friday and then Tuesday and Saturday etc. This will allow the body to recover and grow stronger after each workout.

We replace the power clean with the dead lift and replace the shoulder press with the bench press. We also add weight to leg raises and sit-ups in order to develop the core stability for super strength. Remember that a chain is only as strong as its weakest link.

I recommend increasing your protein intake to slightly over 1 gram per kilogram of body weight, ensure that you eat five types of fruit and vegetables a day or a multivitamin and mineral tablet daily along with a tea spoon of cod liver oil. Cook with olive oil or eat linseed as a snack. This will boost your testosterone, adrenalin and immune system to new heights. These hormones will give you the potential to become super strong.

Weight exercises	Repetitions and sets	Rest
Squats (high bar squats)	10 x 1, 8 x 1, 5 x 4	1 minute
Bench press	10 x 1, 8 x 2	1 minute
Deadlift	10 x 1, 8 x 1, 6 x 2	2 minutes
Pull downs (wide grip)	10 x 1, 8 x 4	1 minute
Sit ups	10 x 3 (8 x 1 with a light weight behind head)	1 minute
Leg raises	10 x 3 (8 x 1 with a light weight between feet)	5 minutes
Stationary Bike ride	15 minutes x 1	1 minute
Calf raises	10 x 2	varied
Stretching back, legs, chest and stomach	5	N/A

FAQS:

1 What exercises should a beginner do?

An absolute beginner should only work with their body weight and get used to lifting their body weight at least 10 times for several sets as outlined in week 1-3 of the program.

2 How often should they train?

Beginners should train every other day. If they trained every day they would burn out, if they trained every three days they would not stimulate enough stress to raise hormone levels to increase adaptations to their body.

3 How long should they train?

They should train for periods between 30 and 60 minutes. A beginner would not be training at a very high intensity and so can afford to train for longer periods.

4 What weights should they use?

Beginners should use both free weights and machines but must limit themselves to light weights for at least three weeks. Beginners should not be straining their bodies, they should be focusing on learning technique and building overall fitness and core stability.

5 What diet should they use?

The diet will depend on whether the lifter intends to get stronger at the same time as gaining, maintaining or loosing weight. The amount of calories should be increased, decreased or maintained based on the weight goals of the beginner.

6 What goals should they set?

Beginners goals for strength should be focused relatively high reps and sets rather than heavy weights. This will prepare them to lift with great intensity when they finally decide to start lifting heavy after the 9th week of the program.

7 Should a beginner have a training partner or be supervised?

With the popularity of websites and online video resources such as Youtube, Vimeo and the like, beginners are attempting to emulate experienced weight trainers lifting amounts and technique or lack of it. Some of the beginners are getting injured before they even get a chance to build any muscle or power.

Most gymnasiums have a policy of induction on how to lift correctly and safely. Some gyms however simply take the membership fee and let the beginner wreck havoc on their bodies. The beginner needs to find someone who is experienced and qualified because some qualified gym instructors only know theories, many of which they have never tried out. What may happen is that the beginner becomes a guinea pig for a program that only works on steroid users and not on natural weight trainers.

Time spent on finding qualified and experienced trainers is time well spent.

8 How does age affect the beginner trainer?

The last quality that a person looses in old age is their strength. There are 60 and even 70 year old power lifters who can bench press over twice their body weight while some 25 year olds can't lift half their body weight. The main contributor to muscular strength is testosterone and tendon strength. Tendon strength is maintained by the collagen protein. This protein normally starts to rapidly decrease after the age of 40. However with scientific advancements and knowledge of diet you can eat special foods which will naturally raise your level of testosterone and content of collagen. A beginner who starts strength training at the age of 50 with the right diet can expect great strength and muscular gains.

9 What is the main reason why beginners give up?

Beginners will quit training normally for one of three reasons:

A: they can't handle the pain of training. B: they become frustrated because they are not seeing the gains quickly enough. C: they feel inadequate they are weak and small in comparison to their peers in the gym. They can overcome this feeling of inadequacy by focusing on their goals and not being distracted by their peers.

10 When is a beginner weight trainer, no longer a beginner?

The beginner advances to another level when he/she knows the technique of lifting weights safely and confidently and have adapted to a weight training program which no longer stresses them to build strength. At this point the strength trainer must assess whether they have achieved their goals and then set new higher level goals.

Chapter 6

Strength training for conditioned athletes

At this intermediate level, lots of sweat and guts are required to take you to the higher echelons of power. An intermediate strength trainer is expected to be able to lift their own body weight in many exercises and should have at least doubled their strength since they started training. The intermediate should have made lots of mistakes and learnt from them. They may have experienced minor injury through over training or errors in technique. All this experience is what should prepare them for super intense strength training with super perfect technique. At this point the strength trainer should know their strength levels and can work on percentages to improve their strength.

In this section it is important for the trainer to increase their calories from root vegetables, and grains, they must eat at least 5 meals a day based on the 1 gram of protein per 1lb of body weight.

At least 2 litres of water must be drunk on non training days and 3 litres drunk on training days.

The body needs to be stressed with different weights and different sets. % = maximum of 1 repetition.

This Intermediate Training Program is done every 4 days alternating heavy deadlifts and squats. Stretching will need to be done every other day to relieve stress and lactic acid.

Intermediate Training Program

Weight exercises	Repetitions and sets	Rest
Squats (low bar squats) Alternating light and heavy with deadlift heavy and light)	10 x 1, 7 x 1, 5 x 1, (light 5 x 60%) (heavy 3 x 80%)	3 minute
Bench press	10 x 1, 8 x 2 (5 x 75% x 3)	1 minute
Deadlift (on light day do heavy squats, on heavy day, light squats)	10 x 1, 8 x 1, 6 x 2, (3 x 75% x 3)	2 minutes
Heave pulls	10 x 1, 8 x 4, (5 x 50% of deadlift max)	1 minute
Sit ups	10 x 1 (8 x 3 heavy weight behind head)	1 minute
Leg raises	10 x 1 (8 x 3 with a heavy weight between feet)	1 minute
Stationary Bike ride	10 minutes x 1	1 minute
Calf raises	10 x 1	varied
Stretching back, legs, chest and stomach	5	N/A

FAQs:

1 How can intermediate weight trainers improve their strength?

They need to work their body into growth and strength with high intensity training and multijoint compound exercises.

2 How do you improve strength without gaining weight?

You must burn more calories and while eating more protein. The calories must come from poly unsaturated fats and a mix complex and simple carbohydrates. Certain fruits and vegetables must be consumed these include: grape fruit, black berries and cranberry juice cucumber, lettuce, celery and tomato.

3 Will weight training for strength make you slow?

It was believed in sport that weight training made you slow however the science and world record holders of track and field have proved this long held belief wrong. The worlds fastest men all use heavy weights in the gym. Tall athletes have found that adding strength to their frame provides the power for them to propel their bodies into a quicker start in the 60 and 100m sprint. Usain Bolt is a classic example of an athlete who was able to transfer a slow start into a world record breaking sprint by using weight training to increase his speed and power.

4 How often should an intermediate weight trainer exercise?

It is better for an intermediate trainer to under train than over train because training at this level of intensity will lead to injury. The strength trainer should check to see if they feel fresh and motivated to train , they should also check the hardness and fullness of their muscles. If their muscles are hard after the previous training session that should mean they have recovered because the body will repair the muscle before attaining its muscle density and hardness.

5 How do you recover from injuries?

If you have any injury normally ice and compression should be applied to stop the swelling of the injury. Depending on the severity of the injury you should start to train around the injury. a pectoral tear or should injury should not stop you training your legs or doing sit ups. This will actually allow you to speed up the recovery of the injured area by increasing blood flow to the whole body.

6 At what age does strength peak?

Looking at the current form of some of the worlds strongest men. Strength seems to peak between 35 and 45 with some strong men competing into their late 50s. A high level of strength can be maintained up to the age of 60 and functional strength can last for the rest of your life if you stay active.

7 What's the best assistance exercise for bench press?

This answer depends on your body type which we saw in chapter 2. Ectomorphs with longer arms tend to benefit from a wider grip and therefore a wide grip pull down would benefit them. Mesomorphs and endomorphs will tend to have shorter arms and therefore benefit from a closer grip bench press which lowers the bar down towards the sternum rather than the upper chest and therefore close grip bench presses and weighted dips can help them.

8 What's the best assistance exercise for the squat?

The squat uses the posterior chain of movement and muscles so the leg press and deadlift would help improve it.

9 What's the best assistance exercise for deadlift?

The same posterior chain is used for the squat and deadlift therefore the lifts are interchangeable. The leg press helps the deadlift a lot for generating the explosiveness to start the lift.

10 How do you stay motivated after many years of training?

You must train in cycles and change your program every 6 to 12 weeks otherwise you get used to the training and stop getting stronger. You also become bored from the lack of mental stimulation.

Chapter 7

Power training for athletes

Sprinters, long jumpers and high jumpers can dramatically improve their performances by doing some very basic movements that involve speed and strength. The athlete will have to increase their protein intake if they want to improve their power. Supplements may assist them if they don't want to add muscular bulk. Whey, hemp or soy protein powder are good quickly absorbed sources of protein.

The power training program for athletes.

Weight exercises	Repetitions and sets	Rest
Speed Squats (high bar squats) slow down fast up)	10 x 1, 7 x 1, 5 x 3 ,	3 minutes
Bench press	10 x 1, 8 x 1 (3 x 60% x 3 sets)	1 minute
Power cleans	10 x 1, 8 x 1, 6 x 2, (3 x 70% x 3 sets)	2 minutes
Heave pulls	10 x 1, 8 x 4, (5 x 100% of power clean max)	1 minute
Sit ups	10 x 1 (8 x 3 with a heavy weight behind head)	1 minute
Leg raises	10 x 1 (8 x 3 sets with a heavy weight between feet)	5 minutes

1 arm overhead kettle bell lifts	10 x 3	1 minute
Calf raises	10 x 3	varied
Stretching back, legs, chest and stomach	7 second holds	N/A

1 How can athletes increase their vertical jump?

They can increase vertical jump by doing fast squats, power cleans and depth jumps where they jump off a box onto the floor and rebound back onto the another or the same box.

2 What's the best power exercise for athletes?

The all-round best exercise for power is the power clean.

3 What's the best power exercise for sprinters?

Again the power clean and clean and jerk.

4 What are the best power exercises for American football or rugby?

The power clean, front squats and low bar back squats, the bench press and overhead press and rows.

5 What is the best power exercise for basket ball?

You can increase your vertical jump by doing fast squats, power cleans and depth jumps where they jump off a box onto the floor and rebound back on a box. Include the bench press and rows for upper body pushing and pulling power.

6 What's the best power exercise for racquet sports?

Dumbbells flys, dumbbell raises, forearm curls, dead lift, squat and kettle bell swings.

7 What's the best power exercise for wrestling?

wide grip and narrow grip rows. Heave pulls and power cleans.

8 What's the best power exercise for boxing?

light dumbbell presses, pull downs, rows, overhead press, push press.

9 Should you strength train before or after aerobic exercise?

When training for strength you need every ounce of creatine and glycogen in your body. Doing aerobic exercise will deplete you of this resource. So it is advised you train aerobically after strength training.

10 How do you recover from strength training as an athlete?

Its very easy to over train so you must take extra protein and multivitamins and minerals, lots of berries and colourful vegetables will help recovery. Take zinc and omega 3 and 6.

Chapter 8

The Bench press

This exercise requires a stable platform to drive the weight off the chest. Assistance exercises will build this base. Always wear a weight lifting belt!

Weight exercises	Repetitions and sets	Rest
Bench press	10 x 1, 7 x 1 , 5 x 5 ,	3 minutes
Overhead press to the back	10 x 1, 8 x 1 6 x 3	1 minute
Dumbbell rows	10 x 1, 8 x 1 , 6 x 2	2 minutes
Shrugs	10 x 1, 8 x 3,	1 minute
Sit ups	10 x 1 (8 x 3 with a heavy weight behind head)	1 minute
Leg raises	10 x 1 (8 x 3 sets with a heavy weight between feet)	5 minutes
1 arm overhead kettle bell lifts	20 x 2	1 minute
Calf raises	10 x 1	Varied
Stretching back, legs, chest and stomach	5 second holds	N/A

Chapter 9

The Squat

This exercise requires stability of the posterior trunk. Because you are squatting heavy you should only do it once a week. The program starts with 70% of maximum weight. Increase the weight by 5% every week.

The Squat program 6 weeks

Weight exercises	Repetitions and sets	Rest
Squats low bar	10 x 1, 8 x 1, 5 x 5,	3 minutes
Leg press	10 x 1, 8 x 1 6 x 3	1 minute
Front squat	10 x 1, 8 x 1, 6 x 3	2 minutes
Box squats from parallel position	10 x 1, 2x 5,	1 minute
Sit ups	10 x 1 (8 x 3 with a heavy weight behind head)	1 minute
Leg raises	10 x 1 (8 x 3 sets with a heavy weight between feet)	5 minutes
Medicine ball waist twists	20 x 2	1 minute
Calf raises	10 x 3	Varied
Stretching back, legs, chest and stomach	5 second holds	N/A

You can improve your strength quite quickly in the squat. Without good technique you can improve the bench press and the deadlift but the squat is unforgiving if you don't have good technique.

If you lift a weight that is too heavy with bad technique in the squat you could be in danger of tearing knee or back ligaments and tendons as well as being crushed by the weight if you don't have good spotters by your side or behind you.

Remember the squat rack is your best friend. Use it as much as possible because if used properly it will minimise your risk of getting injured and greatly improve your strength. Remember always wear a weight lifting belt!

Chapter 10

The Dead lift (The king of the lifts)

This lift requires stability of the upper body and the following program will build great strength in the whole of the body. The program starts with 70% of maximum weight. Increase the weight by 5% every week. Always wear a weight lifting belt! Use the Super strength techniques before starting and practice yoga sun salutation on rest days to aid recovery.

Dead lift program 6 weeks

Weight exercises	Repetitions and sets	Rest
Dead lift	10 x 1, 8 x 1, 5 x 5,	3 minute
Leg press	10 x 1, 8 x 1 6 x 3	1 minute
Heave pulls	10 x 1, 8 x 1, 6 x 3	2 minutes
Pull downs	10 x 1, 2 x 5,	1 minute
Sit ups	10 x 1 (8 x 3 with a heavy weight behind head)	1 minute
Leg raises	10 x 1 (8 x 3 sets with a heavy weight)	5 minutes

Good luck and I wish you a strong and naturally healthy body. Now write down your goals that you want to achieve in 8 weeks in the following exercises. Use the secrets revealed in this book and record your training sessions. For illustrations of exercises please see "The Secrets of Super Strength Illustrated".

Weight exercises	Repetitions and sets	Rest
Squats		1 minute
Bench press		1 minute
Deadlift		2 minutes
Pull downs (wide grip)		1 minute
Power cleans		1 minute
Heave Pulls		5 minutes
Overhead press		1 minute
Weighted sit ups		varied
Stretching back, legs, chest and stomach		N/A

ACKNOWLEDGMENTS

Yoga for you - Tara Fraser - Duncan Baird Publishers 2001).

The Ultimate Book of Martial Arts - Fay Goodman, Hermes House 2003).

The Hypnotic World of Paul Mc Kenna, Boston 1993

. J A Hadfield in the Psychology of power

The human body- a family reference book- Cotton and Adam - Paragon Publishing 2012

Serious Strength Training by Bompa and Di Pasquale

Powerlifting by Austin and Mann

ABOUT THE AUTHOR

Trained in calisthenics from the age of 9. Developed a passion for athletics in track and field. He started weight training at 15 from the teachings of Charles Atlas and much later competed in Powerlifting at county and national level and breaking powerlifting records in the process. He used esoteric methods for developing strength such as yoga, martial arts and psychology to release the full potential of his students.

www.ingramcontent.com/pod-product-compliance
Lightning Source LLC
Chambersburg PA
CBHW070813290526
45795CB00002B/709